MULTIPLE STATEMENT QUESTIONS
IN

Obstetrics and Gynaecology

Part 2

Dr Hakim Gharib Bilal

LIST OF ABBREVIATIONS

ARM	artificial rupture of membranes
BMI	body mass index
BRCA	breast cancer gene
CEA	carcinoembryonic antigen
COCP	combined oral contraceptive pill
CRP	C-reactive protein
CT	computed tomography
ECG	electrocardiography
EDD	expected date of delivery
ESR	erythrocyte sedimentation rate
EUA	examination under anaesthesia
FFP	fresh frozen plasma
FSH	follicle-stimulating hormone
GnRh	gonadotropin releasing hormone
HBA1C	glycosylated haemoglobin
HbF	fetal haemoglobin
hCG	human chorionic gonadotropin
HELLP	haemolysis, elevated liver enzymes and low platelets
HGSIL	high grade squamous intraepithelial lesion
HIV	human immunodeficiency virus
HPV	human papillomavirus
HRT	hormone replacement therapy
HSG	hysterosalpingography
ICSI	intracytoplasmic sperm injection
IUD	intrauterine device
IUGR	intrauterine growth restriction
IUI	intrauterine insemination

LLETZ	large loop excision of transformation zone
LMP	last menstrual period
LGSIL.	low grade squamous intraepithelial lesion
MCMA	monochorionic monoamniotic
MRI	magnetic resonance imaging
MOGTT	modified oral glucose tolerance test
NIDDM	non-insulin dependent diabetes mellitus
OCP	oral contraceptive pill
OHSS	ovarian hyperstimulation syndrome
OGTT	oral glucose tolerance test
PCOS	polycystic ovary syndrome
PCR	polymerase chain reaction
PPH	postpartum haemorrhage
PTT	partial thromboplastin time
PPROM	preterm prelabour rupture of membranes
PROM	prelabour rupture of membranes
RPR	rapid plasma reagin
STI	sexually transmitted infection
SGA	small for gestational age
SLE	systemic lupus erythematosus
TSH	thyroid stimulating hormone
UAE	uterine artery embolisation
UTI	urinary tract infection
VDRL	venereal disease research laboratory
VIN	vulva intraepithelial neoplasia

Acknowledgements:

I would like to express my sincere gratitude to the Dean of the Faculty of Medicine, University Kuala Lumpur Royal College of Medicine Perak, Associate Professor Dr. Syed Rahim, for his unwavering encouragement and moral support throughout this endeavor.

Special appreciation goes to my Head of Department, Associate Professor Dr. Fatehpal Singh Malhi, for his meticulous review, invaluable suggestions, and constructive input that significantly contributed to the refinement of the manuscript.

I extend my heartfelt thanks to my friends and colleagues, particularly Associate Professor Dr. Ariza Mohamed, Dr. Wassim Ahmad, and Professor Dr. Nik Hazlina Nik Hussain from Universiti Sains Malaysia, for their generous assistance in reviewing this manuscript.

Lastly, but certainly not least, I am deeply grateful to my wife and family for their unwavering support and understanding throughout this journey. Their love and encouragement have been my source of strength.

How to Use This Book:

The four statements in each set are straightforward and all focused on providing the same answer. Therefore, if you're unsure of the answer for option A or B, don't give up, as all the questions complement each other. Sometimes, one option alone may be sufficient for you to arrive at the correct answer, while other times, you may need to consider all four options to narrow down to the correct answer.

Think of this process like Global Positioning Satellites (GPS) that work together to pinpoint your location accurately.

Thank you.

1. **Theme:** Types of labour

Statements:

A. This condition describes poor progress of labour.
B. It affects 26% of nulliparous and 8% of multiparous.
C. Usually the labour which was not progressing well stalled at about 6 cm dilatation.
D. Emergency caesarean section is indicated.

Answer	

2. **Theme:** Gynaecological malignancy

Statements:

A. This is the second commonest germ cell tumour.
B. They secrete alpha feto protein.
C. Schiller-Duval body is a defining morphological feature.
D. It has a tendency to spread late, usually to the lungs.

Answer	

3. **Theme:** Drug in Obstetrics

Statements:

A. This belongs to a group of corticosteroids.
B. It should be given to pregnant women between 24 and 34 weeks plus 6 days who are at risk of preterm birth.
C. It accelerates fetal lung maturation.
D. It reduces the risk of necrotising enterocolitis.

Answer	

4. **Theme:** Obstetrics analgesia

Statements:

A. A combination of fentanyl and bupivacaine is used in this procedure.
B. About 1% of patients will experience headache which is made worse by sitting and relieved by lying flat.
C. It is contraindicated in local or systemic sepsis.
D. Maternal hypotension is a possible complication.

Answer	

5. **Theme:** Drugs in Obstetrics

Statements:

    A. This is used in the augmentation of labour.
    B. In combination with ergometrine it is given intramuscularly during the third stage of labour.
    C. Naturally, it is produced by hypothalamus through posterior pituitary gland.
    D. Atociban is an antagonist at the receptor site.

Answer	

6. **Theme:** Drug in gynaecological malignancy

Statements:

    A. This is usually given in combination with carboplatin.
    B. It prevents replication and cell division.
    C. It can cause total loss of all body hair.
    D. It can cause black and tarry stool.

Answer	

7. **Theme:** Reproductive hormone

Statements:

A. This is produced by Leydig cells.
B. In the external genital skin, it is converted into dihydrotestosterone.
C. This is responsible for testicular descent through inguinal canal during early development.
D. A small amount of it is converted into oestradiol in the circulation.

Answer	

8. **Theme:** Investigation of anaemia

Statements:

A. This is a universal intracellular protein that stores iron.
B. The serum level increases during inflammation.
C. This protein is produced by almost all living organisms.
D. It releases iron in a proportionate way.

Answer	

9. **Theme:** Gynaecological malignancy - staging

Statements:

A. Carcinoma confined to the cervix.
B. Can be successfully treated either surgically or by radiotherapy.
C. Radical hysterectomy is a preferred surgical method.
D. Radical trachelectomy is the treatment for young women who have not completed family.

Answer	

10. **Theme:** Obstetrics - risk group

Statements:

A. High risk of postpartum haemorrhage (PPH).
B. A risk factor for utero vaginal prolapse.
C. Risk of uterine rupture.
D. Carries a higher risk of antepartum haemorrhage.

Answer	

11. **Theme:** Gynaecological endocrinology

Statements:

A. This is found in one percent of pregnant women.
B. It may be associated with developmental delay and pregnancy loss.
C. Menstrual irregularity is a possible presenting feature.
D. Levothyroxine is given to patients with this condition.

Answer	

12. **Theme:** Drug in subfertility treatment.

Statements:

A. This has been used in the treatment of breast cancer.
B. This stimulates ovulation.
C. It is an aromatase inhibitor.
D. It works for PCOS.

Answer	

13. **Theme:** Drugs in Obstetrics

Statements:

A. This is used to treat severe postpartum haemorrhage (PPH) due to uterine atony.
B. It can be given intra-myometrium.
C. It is a synthetic prostaglandin analogue PGF2 alpha.
D. It should not be given intravenously.

Answer	

14. **Theme:** Gynaecological malignancy - staging

Statements:

A. Bilateral ovarian tumour with intact capsule.
B. Negative malignant cells in peritoneal fluid.
C. Chemotherapy may be withheld.
D. Overall, 5-year survival is over 90%.

Answer	

15. **Theme:** Obstetrics complication

Statements:

   A. Previous caesarean delivery is a risk factor.
   B. It is associated with a higher risk of maternal morbidity and mortality.
   C. This is present in 80% of patients with placenta praevia.
   D. Ultrasound shows the presence of lacunae and loss of hypoechoic retroplacental space.

Answer	

16. **Theme:** Abnormal labour

Statements:

   A. In this case the progress typically stops or slows after 7cm dilatation.
   B. The possible causes include fetus malposition, malpresentation and cephalopelvic disproportion.
   C. Inadequate uterine contraction is said to be the most common cause.
   D. Caesarean section is advocated.

Answer	

17. **Theme:** Diagnosis in gynaecological condition

Statements:

    A. Ultrasound finding of a cystic mass with ground glass appearance.
    B. Coelomic metaplasia is one of the theories behind it.
    C. CA125 tends to rise.
    D. Diathermy or laser ablation is the treatment of choice for those with subfertility.

Answer	

18. **Theme:** Obstetrics procedure

Statements:

    A. In case of intrauterine death, this is usually done late during labour.
    B. There must be a significant cervical dilatation.
    C. The presenting part must be engaged.
    D. It can shorten the duration of labour.

Answer	

19. **Theme:** Gynaecological malignancy - management

Statements:

    A. This may modify the stage of the tumour.
    B. It may improve the survival rate.
    C. This includes chemotherapy, radiotherapy and hormonal therapy.
    D. In this case chemotherapy is given to shrink the tumour before surgery.

Answer	

20. **Theme**: Multiple pregnancy

Statements:

    A. This condition results from a division of a single fertilised oocyte.
    B. It is the least common type among twins.
    C. It carries a higher perinatal mortality rate due to cord entanglement.
    D. Delivery is by caesarean section at 32-34 weeks' gestation.

Answer	

21. **Theme:**   Infection in pregnancy

Statements:

A. Positive nitrite in urine.
B. The symptoms may be different in pregnancy.
C. The presence of more than 10^5 colony forming units/ml is suggestive.
D. The most common organism involved is E. coli.

Answer	

22. **Theme:** Treatment in postmenopausal condition

Statements:

A. Some patients may experience breast tenderness or swelling.
B. It has a favorable effect on incontinence.
C. It has a favorable effect on sexuality.
D. This is applied locally for patients with vaginal dryness, itching or burning sensation.

Answer	

23. **Theme**: Gynaecological endocrinology

Statements:

A. Testosterone has no effect on sex development.
B. The genitals are entirely female.
C. The complete one may only be diagnosed around the time of puberty.
D. In the case of partial subtype, it can be noticed at birth because the genitals appear different.

Answer	

24. **Theme:** Gynaecological condition.

Statements:

A. This occurs when the columnar cells of the endocervical canal overlie the squamous cells of the ectocervix.
B. It may present as inter-menstrual bleeding.
C. It may develop under the influence of pills.
D. Ablation is one of the treatment modalities.

Answer	

25. **Theme:** Congenital anomaly

Statements:

A. This is due to enzyme deficiency in the production of corticosteroid.
B. 90% is due to 21-hydroxilase enzyme deficiency.
C. There is virilisation of external genitalia due to the raised level of androgen.
D. Two thirds of those with enzyme deficiency will have salt losing variety.

Answer	

26. **Theme:** Gynaecological condition

Statements:

A. This typically occurs late during menstrual cycle.
B. The patient may present with pain or haemorrhage due to rupture.
C. It occurs following ovulation.
D. Expectant management: Analgesia and occasionally laparoscopic surgery may be needed.

Answer	

27. **Theme:** Gynaecological procedure

Statements:

    A. When done posteriorly it can improve obstructed defecation.
    B. Anteriorly it is used to treat cystocele.
    C. It carries a risk of bladder injury.
    D. It may be associated with postoperative dyspareunia.

Answer	

28. **Theme:** Sexually transmitted infection

Statements:

    A. This is a syphilitic ulcer on the genitalia.
    B. It is painless and when the infection has entered the body.
    C. This is the first sign of the infection.
    D. It usually develops three weeks after exposure.

Answer	

29. **Theme:** Gynaecological malignancy

Statements:

    A. These are generally large multiloculated tumours.
    B. Maybe associated with pseudomyxoma peritoneii.
    C. The tumour markers are mostly CA19-9 and CA-125.
    D. Radiologically it has a 'stained glass appearance'.

Answer	

30. **Theme:** Types of ovarian malignancy

Statements:

    A. This occurs mainly in young women.
    B. This is derived from the ovarian primordial germ cells.
    C. This may presents during pregnancy.
    D. Fertility sparing treatment may be preferred.

Answer	

31. **Theme:** Antenatal fetal monitoring.

Statements:

  A. These babies have deficient glycogen stores.
  B. It occurs when estimated fetal weight is less than 10th centile.
  C. Placental insufficiency is the most common cause of this.
  D. In severe cases the umbilical artery doppler may show a reverse end diastolic flow.

Answer	

32. **Theme:** Obstetrics condition

Statements:

  A. This is initially secreted by the amnion.
  B. There is a rapid fall of volume from term onward.
  C. Absence of this in the second trimester is associated with pulmonary hypoplasia.
  D. It contains growth factors and multi-potent stem cells.

Answer	

33. **Theme:** Congenital anomalies.

Statements:

A. This term refers to an abnormal number of chromosomes.
B. Trisomy is the commonest type of this condition.
C. Thickened nuchal fold is one of the soft markers.
D. It may be due to loss or duplication of chromosomes.

Answer	

34. **Theme:** Obstetrics condition

Statements:

A. This is caused by fetal renal agenesis.
B. It may result in pulmonary hypoplasia.
C. Amnioinfusion therapy may improve the outcome in selected patients.
D. Amniotic fluid may be present in significant amounts up to 22 weeks of gestation.

Answer	

35. **Theme:** Drugs in Obstetrics

Statements:

A. This is an oxytocin receptor antagonist.
B. It has similar efficacy to beta sympathomimetics.
C. It is better tolerated.
D. It is the tocolytic agent with the fewest maternal and fetal side effects.

Answer	

36. **Theme:** Early pregnancy condition

Statements:

A. The double ring sign consists of decidua capsularis and decidua parietalis.
B. This can be seen as early as 4 weeks and 1 day.
C. With a blighted ovum, this tends to be empty.
D. In a normal intrauterine pregnancy, this should be visualised by transvaginal scan when beta hCG level is 1500mIU/ml or higher.

Answer	

37. **Theme:** Hormonal treatment in gynaecology

Statements:

A. It lasts for 12 weeks with a two-week grace period.
B. There is a delay in returning to fertility of at least 6 months.
C. It can cause amenorrhoea.
D. There may be 2-3 kg weight gain in the first year of use.

Answer	

38. **Theme:** Congenital abnormality

Statements:

A. This can be reduced by taking folic acid before and during the first weeks of pregnancy.
B. Some of the anti-epileptic medication can increase the risk of this condition.
C. The two most common abnormalities in this condition are anencephaly and spinal bifida.
D. Females are affected more than males.

Answer	

39. **Theme:** Abnormal labour

Statements:

   A. This occurs when the progress of labour which was initially good comes to a halt at 7cm or more.
   B. It can be due to inefficient contraction.
   C. It can be caused by cephalopelvic disproportion.
   D. Caesarean section is the treatment option.

Answer.	

40. **Theme:** Congenital abnormality

Statements:

   A. There is an abdominal wall defect with intestines sticking out.
   B. There is an increased risk of poor fetal growth, decreased amniotic fluid and preterm labour.
   C. In this case there is no sac covering the intestines.
   D. Survival of these infants exceeds 90%.

Answer	

41. **Theme:** Infection in pregnancy

Statements:

    A. Lungs are the most affected organs.
    B. Acyclovir is the drug of choice for this infection.
    C. The maternal mortality rate is five times during pregnancy than non-pregnant condition.
    D. It may cause fetal varicella syndrome.

Answer	

42. **Theme:** Chromosomal abnormality

Statements:

    A. This is caused by a trisomy thirteen.
    B. It is characterised by cleft lip and palate.
    C. Soft markers include echogenic bowel and shortened femur.
    D. The mean survival time is about 130 days.

Answer	

43. Theme: Gynaecological condition

Statements:

A. In this case there is an increase in endometrial gland to stroma ratio.
B. The complex type with atypia is a premalignant condition which may coexist with low grade endometrioid tumour of the endometrium.
C. The risk of progression to endometrial cancer is 25 to 50% for complex with atypia type.
D. The first line of treatment in those without atypia is continuous oral and local (LNG-IUS) progestogens.

Answer	

44. Theme: Obstetrics investigation

Statements:

A. This is a glycoprotein found in cervicovaginal fluid.
B. It is a predictor of preterm delivery.
C. Negative testing has a very high negative predictive value (99.2%).
D. Seventeen percent of women who have a positive test will deliver preterm within two weeks.

Answer	

45. **Theme:** Perinatal infection

Statements:

    A. This is caused by a virus known as Rubivirus.
    B. An infected mother can transmit the infection to her unborn baby by vertical transmission.
    C. The infected baby may have microcephaly, cataract, congenital heart disease and skin rashes.
    D. This can be prevented by MMR vaccine.

Answer	

46. **Theme:** Malpresentation

Statements:

    A. Placenta praevia is a predisposing factor.
    B. There are three types of these conditions.
    C. It occurs in 3 - 4% of all pregnancies at term.
    D. External cephalic version has a success rate of 50-60%.

Answer	

47. **Theme:** Gynaecological anomalies

Statements:

    A. One third of those with this condition have renal anomalies.
    B. Failure of complete canalisation may cause obstruction to menstrual flow.
    C. There may be a complete duplication of the uterus.
    D. In one such condition the patient may present with haematocolpos.

Answer	

48. **Theme:** Obstetrics condition

Statements:

    A. This is one of the causes of traumatic birth and shoulder dystocia.
    B. In this case the fetal weight is 4000 /4500gm or more.
    C. Gestational diabetes mellitus is one of the culprits.
    D. Caesarean section is normally indicated.

Answer	

49. **Theme:** Antenatal complication

statements:

A. It is much more common in preterm fetus.
B. Fetal heart sound is normally detected above maternal umbilicus.
C. A planned vaginal delivery is associated with a 3% increased risk of mortality or morbidity.
D. Mauriceau-Smellie-Veit manoeuvre for delivery of the head if planned vaginal delivery is carried out.

Answer	

50. **Theme:** Perinatal infection

Statements:

A. The B-19 subtype can cause 'slapped cheek' syndrome in children and adults.
B. There is a vertical transmission across the placenta.
C. It can result in hydrops fetalis.
D. About 50% of pregnant women are immune to this virus.

Answer	

51. **Theme:** Normal pregnancy

Statements:

    A. This takes over the endocrine function by the second trimester.
    B. Gushing of blood is a sign of its separation during the third stage.
    C. Inspection upon delivery in case of a missing cotyledon.
    D. Generally, it is one-sixth of the baby's weight.

Answer	

52. **Theme:** Medical disorder in pregnancy

Statements:

    A. This is a preferred treatment for hyperthyroidism in the first trimester.
    B. It may cause liver disease in pregnant women.
    C. Agranulocytosis may develop.
    D. Treatment with this medication increases TSH level.

Answer	

53. **Theme:** Obstetrics complication

Statements:

A. This condition is ten times more common in pregnant than non pregnant woman.
B. Initially they may present with unilateral calf pain or swelling.
C. Low molecular weight heparin is recommended to a high-risk patients.
D. Risk factors include obesity.

Answer	

54. **Theme:** Antenatal care

Statements:

A. This is the measurement from symphysis pubis to the uterine fundus.
B. It has a poor accuracy in determining gestational age.
C. Multiple pregnancy, fetal macrosomia can cause a larger than expected measurement.
D. A uterine fibroid may affect this measurement.

Answer	

55. **Theme:** Perinatal infection

Statements:

    A. Cats are the main reservoir of this infection.
    B. It can cause miscarriage and still birth.
    C. The risk of vertical transmission during the third trimester is higher (60%) compared to the first trimester (15 – 20%).
    D. Ultrasound findings include ventricular dilatation, brain calcification, hepatosplenomegaly and ascites.

Answer	

56. **Theme**: Congenital anomaly

Statements:

    A. About one third of infants with this condition have Down syndrome.
    B. They may present with polyhydramnios.
    C. It is the most common cause of fetal bowel obstruction.
    D. Ultrasound shows a 'double bubble' sign.

Answer	

57. **Theme:** Obstetrics condition

Statements:

A. There is an unequal blood flow between twins.
B. It occurs in monochorionic twins.
C. Can be confirmed by comparing middle cerebral artery blood flow between the twins.
D. Fetal demise may occur, donors are more likely to be affected than the recipient.

Answer	

58. **Theme:** Antenatal fetal monitoring

Statements:

A. This is the most sensitive biometric measurement for predicting intrauterine growth restriction.
B. In fetal growth restriction it tends to cross the centile in a serial ultrasound scan.
C. In large for gestation fetus, it crosses the 95th centile.
D. It is not as accurate as other parameters in measuring gestational age.

Answer	

59. **Theme:** Early pregnancy structure

Statements:

  A. This is the primary source of exchange between mother and fetus in early pregnancy.
  B. It is the first embryonic structure to be visualized sonographically.
  C. It should be visualized by five weeks by transvaginal scan when the gestational sac is 8 mm or more.
  D. It gives a good overview of pregnancy outcome in the first trimester.

Answer	

60. **Theme:** Antenatal fetal monitoring

Statements:

  A. This shows the interval between successive fetal heartbeats.
  B. It is reduced in case of fetal sleep states, opioid use or fetal hypoxia.
  C. A normal value reflects normal fetal autonomic nervous system.
  D. It increases with increasing gestational age.

Answer	

61. **Theme:** Gynaecological procedure

Statements:

    A. This is used in tubal patency test.
    B. This is used in undiagnosed pelvic pain.
    C. This is used in suspected ectopic pregnancy.
    D. This is used in female sterilisation.

Answer	

62. **Theme:** Drug in gynaecology

Statements:

    A. This has an antioestrogenic effect at a higher level.
    B. This acts on pituitary and hypothalamus.
    C. This leads to an increase in FSH and LH production.
    D. Its usage can lead to twin pregnancy.

Answer	

63. **Theme:** Fetal monitoring

Statements:

  A. The baseline tends to fall with advancing gestation age.
  B. The normal range is 110 – 150 beats per minute.
  C. It goes above normal in case of maternal fever or fetal hypoxia.
  D. Drugs such as beta adrenoceptor agonist can increase the range.

Answer	

64. **Theme:** Drugs in gynaecology

Statements:

  A. This reduces heavy menstrual loss by 30%.
  B. This aids in dysmenorrhea.
  C. It is advised to take it with food.
  D. It can cause gastrointestinal bleeding.

Answer	

65. **Theme:** Enzyme deficiency in gynaecological condition

Statements:

   A. It affects male sexual development.
   B. They are genetically male.
   C. This converts testosterone into dihydrotestosterone.
   D. There is an increasing virilisation of a female child during puberty due to increased circulation of testosterone.

Answer	

66. **Theme:** Drug in gynaecology

Statements:

   A. This is a synthetic steroid.
   B. This conserves bone mass.
   C. This improves libido.
   D. This is used with long term GnRH analogues to preserve bone strength.

Answer	

67. **Theme:** Gynaecological condition

Statements:

    A. This is usually diagnosed when the cyst measures more than 3 cm.
    B. It includes follicular, corpus luteal and theca luteal cyst.
    C. They usually go away without treatment.
    D. Combined oral contraceptive pill reduces the risk.

Answer	

68. **Theme:** Gynaecological examination

Statements:

    A. Abdominal mass less than 12 weeks of pregnancy can be assessed.
    B. Tenderness on cervical motion can be assessed.
    C. A lesion or scaring of uterosacral ligament can be appreciated.
    D. Adnexal mass can be better examined.

Answer	

69. **Theme:** Hormonal contraceptive device

Statements:

   A. This reduces heavy menstrual bleeding by 90% in twelve months.

   B. It is effective for treating secondary dysmenorrhoea.

   C. It protects endometrium against hyperplasia.

   D. Once removed, return to fertility is not delayed.

Answer	

70. **Theme:** Gynaecological procedure

Statements:

   A. This used to be a primary procedure for stress incontinence.

   B. This is an open abdominal procedure.

   C. The cure rate is 80 – 85%.

   D. It carries a risk of posterior vaginal prolapse.

Answer	

71. **Theme:** Gynaecological condition

Statements:

    A. Ultrasound may show haematocolpos with or without haematometra.
    B. The patient may present with urinary symptoms/ retention.
    C. Primary amenorrhoea is a presenting complain.
    D. Surgical therapy (hymenotomy, hymenectomy) is the recommended treatment option.

Answer	

72. **Theme:** Infection in Gynaecology

Statements:

    A. These are vaginal cells that appear fuzzy under microscope without sharp edges.
    B. A vaginal pH of 4.5 or higher.
    C. A group of Gram-variable bacteria is responsible for this condition.
    D. Douching is a risk factor.

Answer	

73. **Theme:** Benign gynaecological tumour

Statements:

    A. This tumour is composed only of dermal and epidermal elements.
    B. It is also known as matured cystic teratoma.
    C. Most of them are benign.
    D. It can contain skin appendage, teeth and hair follicles.

Answer	

74. **Theme:** Drug in gynaecology

Statements:

    A. This has an androgenic effect.
    B. It has suppressing effect on ovarian function.
    C. It had been used in the management of endometriosis and abnormal per vaginal bleeding.
    D. Due to its side effect, the drug was discontinued in some countries.

Answer	

75. **Theme:** Gynaecological procedure

Statements:

A. This destroys the endometrial layer.
B. Indicated for abnormal uterine bleeding.
C. Contraindicated in endometrial hyperplasia or uterine malignancy.
D. It can result in uterine perforation.

Answer	

76. **Theme:** Benign gynaecological condition

Statements:

A. The patient may present with intermenstrual bleeding.
B. It can be pedunculated.
C. They are usually benign (1% may show malignant transformation).
D. Hysteroscopic removal is the recommended treatment option.

Answer	

77. **Theme:** Gynaecological condition

Statements:

A. It has a ground glass appearance on ultrasound, a feature which is also seen in haemorrhagic cyst.
B. This contains a thick dark brown fluid.
C. Its presence indicates a more severe disease state (stage III or IV).
D. Laparoscopy is the gold standard for diagnosis and treatment.

Answer	

78. **Theme:** Gynaecological condition

Statements:

A. This is caused by increased exposure of cervical epithelium to oestrogen.
B. It is common in women who are taking oral contraceptive pills.
C. It is a common finding in pregnancy.
D. It can cause post coital or intermenstrual bleeding.

Answer	

79. **Theme:** Gynaecological condition

Statements:

A. This has been associated with endometrioid or clear cell type of ovarian cancer.
B. Patients with this condition have elevated level of pro-inflammatory cytokines (IL1, IL6 and IL8).
C. Laparoscopically the lesion can appear as red, 'matchstick' or white and fibrous.
D. Medical treatment does not improve fertility.

Answer	

80. **Theme:** Hormonal contraception

Statements:

A. This has little effect on ovarian activity.
B. It causes endometrial atrophy.
C Contains levonorgestrel.
D. It does not prevent ovulation.

Answer	

81. **Theme:** Obstetrics procedure

Statements:

A. This is done during caesarean section.
B. Placenta accreta spectrum is one of the indications.
C. Can be done due to life threatening maternal haemorrhage.
D. It is indicated for uterine atony which is not responding to uterotonic drugs.

Answer	

82. **Theme:** Gynaecological malignancy - staging

Statements:

A. Radical hysterectomy with bilateral lymph node dissection is the standard treatment.
B. Radical trachelectomy and bilateral node dissection for those who want to retain fertility.
C. In the early part of this stage, pelvic radiotherapy has a similar success rate to surgery.
D. Clinical lesion confined to the cervix.

Answer	

83. **Theme:** Gynaecological condition.

Statements:

    A. This reflects a chronic manifestation of pelvic inflammatory disease (PID).
    B. There is a right upper quadrant pain.
    C. It involves inflammation of liver capsule.
    D. Violin-string adhesion between the liver and abdominal wall or diaphragm can be seen during laparoscopy.

Answer	

84. **Theme:** Gynaecological infection

Statements:

    A. This is a Gram-variable bacillus.
    B. This is considered as a key pathogen in bacterial vaginosis.
    C. It is part of vaginal flora.
    D. It can be treated with clindamycin and metronidazole.

Answer	

85. **Theme:** Gynaecological malignancy

Statements:

A. Recurrence can occur years after the primary has been treated.
B. Over 80% are bilateral.
C. Ovarian metastasis associated with primary cancers of the colon, breast and stomach.
D. The patients may have a positive cytokeratin, elevated CEA or CA125.

Answer	

86. **Theme**: Pain in gynaecology

Statements:

A. This is described as deep and superficial.
B. This can be caused by endometriosis or pelvic inflammatory disease.
C. It is characterised by discomfort, burning or throbbing pain during intercourse.
D. Topical oestrogen application is one of the treatment options for those with atrophic vaginitis.

Answer	

87. **Theme:** Congenital anomaly

Statements:

  A. This is an X-linked recessive condition.
  B. The deficiency in GnRH results in underdeveloped genitalia.
  C. The patient may have a delayed or absent puberty with impaired sense of smell.
  D. It is a form of hypogonadotropic hypogonadism.

Answer	

88. **Theme:** Gynaecological procedure

Statements:

  A. This procedure can induce ovulation in patients with PCOS.
  B. Indicated for those who have not responded to medical treatment (Clomiphene citrate).
  C. About 50% pregnancy rate after the procedure.
  D. The mean anti-mullerian hormone (AMH) level decreases significantly after this procedure.

Answer	

89. **Theme:** Gynaecological condition

Statements:

   A. In this there is a hereditary predisposition to colon, endometrial and ovarian cancer.

   B. It runs in families in an autosomal dominant inheritance pattern.

   C. This is suspected when three or more family members have related cancers.

   D. There are two types of this condition; endometrial cancer occurs in type 1 of this condition.

Answer	

90. **Theme:** Gynaecological malignancy

Statements:

   A. This is an androgen producing tumour.

   B. Patients may present with abdominal mass and signs of virilization.

   C. Surgery is the mainstay of treatment as there is no effective chemotherapy for this condition.

   D. Twenty five percent are malignant.

Answer	

91. **Theme:** Drug in Obstetrics.

Statements:

   A. This drug has no teratogenic effect.
   B. In the body it is metabolized to alpha methyl norepinephrine which is an active metabolite.
   C. It can make direct Coombs test positive.
   D. It is a centrally acting antihypertensive.

Answer	

92. **Theme:** Gynaecological malignancy

Statements:

   A. This behaves similarly to serous ovarian cancer.
   B. It is classed as stage 3 or 4 and mestastasis as stage 4.
   C. In this condition there is a tendency to have a normal sized or slightly bulky ovaries.
   D. There is more of an extra ovarian disease than the actual ovarian problem.

Answer	

93. **Theme:** Factors that prevent against this cancer

Statements:

- A. Combined oral contraceptive pill.
- B. Pregnancy.
- C. Smoking.
- D. Hysterectomy.

Answer	

94. **Theme:** Gynaecological investigation

Statements:

- A. It is indicated in patients with urge, stress and neurological urinary incontinence.
- B. In this case the patient needs to complete a 3-day bladder diary.
- C. It can be complicated by urinary tract infection.
- D. It is the gold standard for assessing urinary symptoms.

Answer	

95. **Theme:** Staging in gynaecological condition

Statements:

   A. This is a sexual maturity rating.
   B. It is used to assess pubertal development.
   C. Menarche typically occurs at stage 4 breast development.
   D. In stage 5 there is mature adult breast.

Answer	

96. **Theme:** Gynaecological condition

Statements:

   A. This is described as burning pain sensation.
   B. It occurs without skin disease or infection.
   C. Typically, the pain last for three months or more.
   D. Neuromodulators such as tricyclic antidepressants are of limited benefit.

Answer	

97. **Theme:** Hormone in gynaecology.

Statements:

    A. It is given in place of LH during IVF cycle.
    B. Blood or protein in urine may cause false positive results.
    C. "Hook effect", when hCG level is about 500 000mIU/mL. can cause false serum negative.
    D. The maximum hormonal level is reached by 10 weeks of pregnancy.

Answer	

98. **Theme:** Gynaecological malignancy

Statements:

    A. Human Papilloma Virus infection has been implicated.
    B. The less common one is associated with skin condition such as lichen sclerosis.
    C. This is a precancerous condition.
    D. It can present with itching, burning, tingling or soreness in the vulval area.

Answer	

99. **Theme:** Hormones in Obstetrics and Gynaecology

Statements:

A. It is the dominant hormone after ovulation.
B. Mifepristone is an antagonist to this hormone.
C. It peaks to 35-50nmol/L in mid luteal phase.
D. It is responsible for implantation and maintenance of pregnancy.

Answer	

100. **Theme:** Obstetrics investigation

Statements:

A. In patients with anaemia, sickle cell disease or G6PD, it may appear as false "good" result.
B. American diabetes association has recently recommended this as a diagnostic criteria for diabetes mellitus with a cut-point of >/= 6.5% as an alternative to fasting blood glucose.
C. In pregnancy MOGTT is a preferred test than this.
D. Range in non-diabetics is 4-5.6%.

Answer	

101. **Theme:** Hormones in Obstetrics and gynaecology

Statements:

    A. This is one of the three types of oestrogen.
    B. It is the weakest of them.
    C. It is primarily present during pregnancy.
    D. During pregnancy the level increases 1000-fold as compared to the other types (100-fold).

Answer	

102. **Theme**: Drug in Obstetrics and Gynaecology

Statements:

    A. This is used to treat hyperprolactinaemia.
    B. It is usually given twice a week for at least 6 months.
    C. For breast milk suppression only one dose is given (0.5mg).
    D. It is a potent dopamine receptor agonist.

Answer	

103. **Theme:** Maternal mortality

Statements:

    A. This occurs from causes that are not related to pregnancy.
    B. This involves motor vehicle accident.
    C. Suicide or violent death are included in this category.
    D. Also termed as 'coincidental'.

Answer	

104. **Theme:** Assessment in Obstetrics and gynaecology

Statements:

    A. This is an important landmark in clinical pelvic assessment.
    B. The shortest distance from pubic symphysis to this area is 11.5cm.
    C. It is prominent in an android pelvis.
    D. Diagonal conjugate is measured from the lower border of symphysis pubis to this area.

Answer	

105. **Theme:** Assessment in Obstetrics and Gynaecology

Statements:

A. This is an important landmark in obstetrics examination.
B. The fetal head is said to be in station zero when the lower part of fetal head is at this level.
C. When prominent the pelvic size maybe inadequate.
D. It is located in the narrowest part of the pelvis.

Answer	

106. **Theme:** Type of contraception

Statements:

A. This is a permanent contraceptive method.
B. Semen analysis is advised after three months of the procedure.
C. It is done under local anaesthesia.
D. It is considered as the safest with least complications.

Answer	

107. **Theme:** Abnormal uterine bleeding

Statements:

   A. This is a common concern among women taking hormonal contraceptive method.
   B. It is a bleeding which occurs between menstrual periods.
   C. The most frequent is progestin induced.
   D. Management includes counselling and reassurance as well as supplemental oestrogen (in patients with progestin only medication).

Answer	

108. **Theme**: Abnormal vaginal bleeding

Statements:

   A. This can be caused by cancer or precancerous condition of uterus or cervix.
   B. It can be caused by Chlamydia infection.
   C. Often seen with endometrial and cervical polyp.
   D. It is also known as bleeding between periods.

Answer	

109. **Theme:** Drug in Obstetrics and gynaecology

Statements:

A. This is a macrolide antibiotic.
B. It is bacteriostatic.
C. It is effective against Chlamydia.
D. It is recommended for prophylaxis in PPROM.

Answer	

110. **Theme:** Drug in obstetrics

Statements:

A. This is given to reduce methotrexate side effects.
B. It is used to treat megaloblastic anaemia.
C. It helps prevent neural tube defects.
D. The recommended dose for women of reproductive age is 400mcg daily.

Answer	

111. **Theme:** Drug in gynaecology

Statements:

- A. This lowers the testosterone level in the body.
- B. It is used to treat hirsutism.
- C. Combined with ethinyl estradiol, it is used as a combined oral contraceptive pill.
- D. It has been used to treat prostate cancer.

Answer	

112. **Theme:** Obstetrics monitoring

Statements:

- A. This is a blood-stained mucus.
- B. This may appear around the onset of labour.
- C. Normally it is about 1 to 2 tablespoons.
- D. If excessive it can be mistaken for antepartum haemorrhage.

Answer	

113. **Theme:** Gynaecological malignancy

Statements:

A. This is inherited in an autosomal dominant manner.
B. Risk factors include family history of breast cancer at or before the age of 50 years.
C. Apart from breast cancer, it typically involves epithelial ovarian cancer, fallopian tube cancer and primary peritoneal cancer.
D. A parent has a 50% chance of passing the gene to the offspring.

Answer	

114. **Theme:** Contraceptive method

Statements:

A. This contains etonogestrel.
B. It is radio opaque as it contains Barium.
C. It is implanted subdermal.
D. Effective for three years.

Answer	Nexplanon

115. **Theme:** Obstretrics and gynaecological examination

Statements:

    A. This is used to confirm the leaking liquor.
    B. This is used to examine the cervix.
    C. This is used to find the source of vaginal bleeding.
    D. This is used during cervical smear.

Answer	

116. **Theme:** Labour

Statements:

    A. When the fetus is delivered in less than three hours of the commencement of regular contractions.
    B. It can result in a ruptured uterus.
    C. It is a risk factor for postpartum haemorrhage.
    D. It can cause fetal hypoxia.

Answer	

117. **Theme:** Obstetrics condition

Statements:

A. This is a benign tumour of the placenta arising from chorionic tissue.
B. This can result in hydrops fetalis.
C. This can result in polyhydramnios.
D. It can be treated by laser ablation of feeding vessels.

Answer	

118. **Theme:** Drug in Obstetrics

Statements:

A. This is given to treat hypocalcemia.
B. It must be given slowly to avoid venous damage and prevent syncopal attack possibly due to high concentration of calcium reaching the heart.
C. It is used to treat cardiac toxicity due to hyperkalaemia.
D. It is used as an antidote for magnesium sulphate toxicity.

Answer	

119. **Theme:** Hormone in gynaecology

Statements:

  A. This is one of three types of estrogens made by the body.
  B. It is the weak type of oestrogen.
  C. The level is typically higher after menopause.
  D. It is produced by ovaries, adipose tissues and adrenal glands.

Answer	

120. **Theme:** Antenatal condition

Statements:

  A. This is the normal finding before 37 weeks.
  B. Placenta praevia is a risk factor.
  C. Fetal lie chart is normally used as a monitoring tool.
  D. Cord prolapse is a possible complication.

Answer	

121. **Theme:** Puerperal complication

Statements:

A. This is a transient self-limited low mood and depressive symptoms.
B. It occurs mainly between the first and tenth day postpartum.
C. It lasts up to two weeks.
D. It is caused by hormonal changes after delivery.

Answer	

122. **Theme:** Malignancy in Obstetrics and gynaecology

Questions:

A. The presence of paternal DNA distinguishes gestational from non-gestational.
B. A fast-growing malignant tumour that arises from trophoblastic cells.
C. It commonly spreads to the lungs.
D. It can also occur in male.

Answer	

123. **Theme**: Obstetrics investigation

Questions:

    A. This is commonly elevated in women with preeclampsia.
    B. Increased level correlates with an adverse fetal outcome in patients with preeclampsia.
    C. The increased level precedes hypertension and proteinuria.
    D. Serum level tends to be higher in men and postmenopausal women.

Answer	

124. **Theme:** Tumour marker

Statements:

    A. The level of this is elevated in colorectal, prostate, breast and ovarian mucinous cystadenocarcinoma.
    B. Hence a nonspecific tumour marker.
    C. The serum level may rise when taking antineoplastic drugs such as 5-fluorouracil.
    D. Smoking and aging increase the level.

Answer	

125. **Theme:** Investigation in Obstetrics

Statements:

   A. This test looks for the antibodies present in maternal blood.
   B. A negative test implies that the fetus is not in danger of being attacked by maternal Rhesus antibodies.
   C. It tends to be negative for those given anti D immunoglobulin prophylaxis.
   D. It is done if there is blood transfusion reaction.

Answer	

126. **Theme:** Gynaecological condition

Statements:

   A. This is a skin condition with dark discolouration around the body folds.
   B. It is caused by insulin resistance.
   C. It is a common feature in patients with polycystic ovarian syndrome.
   D. It disappears once the cause is treated.

Answer	

127. **Theme:** Fetal anomaly

Questions:

A. Presence of double bubble sign on ultrasound image.
B. This may cause bilious or non-bilious vomiting during the first 24 to 38 hours after birth.
C. The mother may present with polyhydramnios.
D. 30 to 40% of children with this condition have Down syndrome.

Answer	

128. **Theme:** Management in urogynaecological condition.

Statements:

A. It can improve incontinence.
B. It has been found to improve sexual function.
C. It can help with pelvic organ prolapse.
D. This is a pelvic floor muscle exercise.

Answer	

129. **Theme:** Monitoring in Obstetrics

Statements:

A. Absence of this in the second trimester can cause pulmonary hypoplasia.
B. It is reduced in cases of placental insufficiency.
C. It cushions the growing fetus.
D. When left to dry in a glass it crystalizes in a fern like pattern.

Answer	

130. **Theme:** Gynaecological tumour

Questions:

A. They are usually diagnosed during reproductive age.
B. In this case there is an abnormal mitotic activity with no stromal invasion.
C. TAHBSO has been the mainstay of the treatment, however, fertility-sparing surgery could be a valid option for women desiring fertility.
D. In this case the usage of CA 125 is controversial.

Answer	

131. **Theme:** Cardiac disorder in pregnancy

Statements:

    A. This is a cyanotic heart disease.
    B. There is pulmonary hypertension.
    C. Deoxygenated blood bypasses the lungs and enters general circulation.
    D. Pregnancy is contraindicated.

Answer	

132. **Theme:** Antenatal monitoring

Statements:

    A. Abdominal inspection shows distended flanks.
    B. The fetal poles may be felt on either side of maternal abdomen.
    C. Pelvic grip may be felt "empty".
    D. Placenta praevia, fetal and uterine abnormalities are some of the known risk factors.

Answer	

133. **Theme:** Obstetrics condition

Statements:

  A. This happened in monochorionic monoamniotic twin.
  B. The most common type is thoraco-omphalopagus.
  C. The ratio of female to male is 3 to 1.
  D. This happens when separation occurs more than 13 days after fertilization.

Answer	

134. **Theme:** Female reproductive system

Statements:

  A. In patients with severe endometriosis the uterus can be bound down by dense adhesions in this position.
  B. This occurs in one fifth of women.
  C. Most women are asymptomatic.
  D. If this condition is missed, there is a risk of perforation through the anterior wall with surgical instruments.

Answer	

135. **Theme:** Management in gynaecological malignancy

Statements:

    A. This can be delivered as teletherapy or brachytherapy.
    B. Selenium is used as one of the sources of treatment for this modality.
    C. The patient may need to undergo examination under anaesthesia.
    D. The cure rate may increase when given in combination with chemotherapy such as cisplatin.

Answer	

136. **Theme:** Pelvic drainage

Statements:

    A. This is divided into superficial and deep.
    B. They drain anal canal, vulva, and clitoris.
    C. They drain into external iliac nodes.
    D. They become tender, ulcerated with exudate in patients with *Haemophilus ducreyi* infection.

Answer	

137. **Theme:** Management in Obstetrics complication

Statements:

    A. This is given when there is an abnormal coagulation test.
    B. It is given to reverse the effect of warfarin in the presence of active bleeding.
    C. It may not be tolerated in patients with liver disease.
    D. It is free of red and white blood cells.

Answer	

138. **Theme:** Lymphatic drainage in gynaecological malignancy

Statements:

    A. These are located along the internal iliac arteries.
    B. They receive drainage from upper vagina, cervix and the body of the uterus.
    C. They drain to common iliac and para-aortic lymph nodes.
    D. They used to be known as hypogastric nodes.

Answer	

139. Theme: Obstetrics investigation finding

Statements:

   A. This is one of the cardinal features of pre-eclampsia.
   B. When 300mg or more per 24 hours, it is considered as pre-eclampsia.
   C. It can occur in patients with primary kidney disease.
   D. Foamy urine is widely regarded as a sign of this.

Answer	

140. Theme: Female reproductive system

Statements:

   A. This part of the endometrium forms a placental base.
   B. It consists of three layers.
   C. Part of it forms the maternal component of the placenta.
   D. It supports embryo development prior to placenta formation.

Answer	

141. **Theme:** Finding in gynaecological procedure

Statements:

   A. This is used to describe HPV transient infection related changes.
   B. A major identifiable feature of this is koilocytosis.
   C. The risk of cervical cancer is less than 1 percent.
   D. It is generally considered as mild dysplasia.

Answer	

142. **Theme:** Assisted reproductive technique

Statements:

   A. Ovarian hyperstimulation syndrome is a possible complication.
   B. In some patients with male sub-fertility, intracytoplasmic sperm injection is needed.
   C. Multiple pregnancies are a possible outcome.
   D. Tubal factor subfertility is a common indication.

Answer	

143. **Theme:** Gynaecological malignancy

Statements:

A. This is considered as moderate or severe cervical dysplasia.
B. The risk of cervical cancer is as high as 7%.
C. HPV is a major aetiological agent.
D. Colposcopy may show dense acetowhite epithelium.

Answer	

144. **Theme:** Types of labour

Statements:

A. Time between the onset of painful uterine contractions and cervical dilatation of 4 cm.
B. During this time the cervix becomes fully effaced.
C. It lasts between 3 to 8hours.
D. It is shorter in multiprous.

Answer	

145. **Theme:** Drug in gynaecology

Statements:

    A. This is a depot preparation which is given subdermally.
    B. It is used in the management of fibroids and endometriosis.
    C. Long term use can cause loss of bone mineral density.
    D. It is a gonadotropin-releasing hormone agonist.

Answer	

146. **Theme:** Urogynaecological anomalies

Statements:

    A. There is an embryologic growth failure of mullerian duct.
    B. There is an absence or hypoplasia of vagina.
    C. There is normal ovarian, breast and pubic hair development.
    D. Presents with primary amenorrhoea.

Answer	

147. **Theme:** Complication of Gynaecological condition

Statements:

    A. This can lead to endometrial hyperplasia or carcinoma.
    B. Diabetes mellitus due to insulin resistance.
    C. Hypertension and cardiovascular disease.
    D. Infertility is due to hyperandrogenism which leads to anovulation.

Answer	

148. **Theme:** Gynaecological endocrine condition.

Statements:

    A. This involves the cessation of periods before 40 years old.
    B. It involves 1% of women under 40years.
    C. It can be caused by chromosomal abnormalities such as Fragile X.
    D. It can be caused by chemotherapy, radiotherapy or infection such as Mump virus.

Answer	

149. **Theme:** Medical condition in Obstetrics

Statements:

A. When exposed to sunlight it can result in skin rashes and flares.
B. Antinuclear antibody test is usually an initial test.
C. There is an increased risk of early miscarriage, nephritis and pre-eclampsia.
D. The fetus is at risk of congenital heart block.

Answer	

150. **Theme:** Anatomy of female genital track

Statements:

A. The position of this varies throughout life.
B. The area between the new and old position is transformation zone.
C. When there is an overlying of squamous and columnar epithelium nabothian follicle is formed.
D. This is where the two types of epitheliums meet.

Answer	

151. **Theme:** Hormone in gynaecology

Statements:

A. This suppresses ovarian activity and results in amenorrhoea.
B. Patients may present with features of hypoestrogenism such as vaginal dryness.
C. About 80% will respond to dopamine agonist treatment.
D. Some patients may need trans-sphenoidal adenectomy.

Answer	

152. **Theme:** Gynaecological malignancy

Statements:

A. This is associated with Hereditary Non-Polyposis Colorectal Cancer Syndrome.
B. Cervical smear may show abnormal glandular cytology.
C. High grade serous and clear cell subtypes have the worst prognosis.
D. The type one has characteristic growth factor alteration.

Answer	

153. **Theme:** Gynaecological malignancy

Statements:

A. The Human epididymis protein 4 test is positive.
B. The usage of combined oral contraceptive pills provides some protection.
C. Nulliparity is a risk factor.
D. Tumour markers include CA 125, CA 19-9, CEA.

Answer	

154. **Theme:** Investigation in Obstetrics

Statements:

A. This is a glycoprotein found in cervico-vaginal fluid, amniotic fluid and placental tissue.
B. It's presence in cervico-vaginal fluid between 22 to 36 weeks is a good predictor of preterm delivery.
C. It has a very high negative predictive value.
D. Digital examination and prior speculum examination may result in false positive results.

Answer	

155. **Theme:** Benign gynaecological condition

Statements:

    A. This is commonly associated with twins or molar pregnancy.
    B. The cyst is often bilateral.
    C. It is also termed as hyperreactio luteinalis.
    D. Most of them resolve spontaneously during pregnancy.

Answer	

156. **Theme:** Anatomy of female reproductive system

Statements:

    A. This is an area of squamous metaplasia.
    B. Premalignancy and malignancy tend to develop here.
    C. It must be visualised during colposcopic examination.
    D. HPV infection can trigger oncogenic processes in this area.

Answer	

157. **Theme:** Hormones in gynaecology

Statements:

   A. This is produced by growing follicles in the ovary.
   B. It plays a role in male sex differentiation.
   C. It is used to assess functional ovarian reserve.
   D. It is measured during the early follicular phase.

Answer	

158. **Theme:** Medical disorder in pregnancy

Statements:

   A. This doesn't cross the placenta.
   B. This is stopped soon after the delivery of the baby by a gestational diabetic mellitus mother.
   C. It can cause lipodystrophy.
   D. Patients with uncontrolled early morning blood glucose are given intermediate acting preparation.

Answer	

159. **Theme:** Drug in gynaecology

Statements:

    A. It is used in the management of prostate cancer.
    B. Its maximum usable duration is 6 months.
    C. It is used to treat precocious puberty in children.
    D. Given 4 weekly Intramuscularly, it is used to reduce uterine fibroid size.

Answer	

160. **Theme:** Haematological products in Obstetrics and gynaecology

Statements:

    A. This has a shelf life of 5 days at room temperature.
    B. Spleen acts as a reservoir.
    C. This is used to support patients with severe thrombocytopaenia and as part of massive blood transfusion.
    D. They don't need crossmatching.

Answer	

161. **Theme:** Antenatal fetal monitoring

Statements:

A. This is used to calculate percentile size for a given gestation.
B. This chart is based on ultrasound measurement.
C. With this tool a measurement of less than 10th centile is considered as small for gestation.
D. A measurement of more than 90th centile is considered as large for gestation.

Answer	

162. **Theme:** Drug in Obstetrics and gynaecology.

Statements:

A. This is used for anaerobes.
B. It has a characteristic metallic taste.
C. It is used in the treatment of bacterial vaginosis.
D. It crosses the blood brain barrier.

Answer	

163. **Theme:** Early pregnancy complication

Statements:

    A. It has been associated with high beta hCG level.
    B. Multiple pregnancy is a risk factor.
    C. It is a diagnosis of exclusion.
    D. It subsides by the second trimester.

Answer	

164. **Theme:** Urogynaecological condition

Statements:

    A. Forward protrusion of urinary bladder bulging the anterior wall of the vagina
    B. The patient may present with urinary incontinence.
    C. Risk factors include multiparity.
    D. Pelvic floor exercise is one of the treatment modalities.

Answer	

165. **Theme:** Haematological preparation in Obstetrics and gynaecology

Statements:

A. This has a shelf life of one year.
B. It contains all the clotting factors.
C. It must be ABO compatible. (Crossmatch is not required).
D. It is indicated in situations where clotting factors are deficient.

Answer	

166. **Theme:** Haematology in Obstetrics and gynaecology

Statements:

A. This is a fibrinogen rich protein with Factor VIII and von Willebrand factor.
B. It should be compatible with the ABO blood group of the patient.
C. It is used as part of the Disseminated Intravascular Coagulation (DIC) regime.
D. It has been used to treat von Willebrand's disease and haemophilia.

Answer	

167. **Theme:** congenital defect

Statements:

A. This may be associated with fetal genetic defects and other anomalies.
B. It has an association with Beckwith-Wiedemann syndrome (one third).
C. There is a herniation of abdominal organs through a central abdominal wall defect covered by peritoneum and amnion.
D. It can be detected by ultrasound from 14 weeks of gestation.

Answer	

168. **Theme:** Infection in Obstetrics

Statements:

A. Ruptured membranes are a risk factor.
B. To prevent the infection, antibiotics are recommended after 18 hours of leaking.
C. It can result in a bad obstetrics outcome.
D. It can present with fever, abdominal pain and change in liquor colour.

Answer	

169. **Theme:** Gynaecological infection

Statements:

   A. Type 6 and 11 are associated with condylomata acuminata.
   B. Verruca vulgaris or verruca plantaris are caused by subtype 1,2,4 and 27.
   C. Multiple partners is a risk factor.
   D. Subtypes 16 and 18 are responsible for cervical malignancy.

Answer	

170. **Theme:** Anatomy of the peritoneal cavity

Statements:

   A. This helps in the control of local infection.
   B. It is a fat storage layer.
   C. It contains "milky spots" that contribute to the organ's immune function.
   D. Part of this structure is dissected in the management and staging of ovarian cancer.

Answer	

171. **Theme:** Post menopausal complication

Statements:

    A. Soy isoflavones can provide some relief for this condition.
    B. Selective serotonin inhibitors are helpful for patients who cannot take hormones.
    C. Fezolinetant is a recently approved medication for this condition.
    D. It can persist for two to four years after menopause.

Answer	

172. **Theme:** Antenatal monitoring

Statements:

    A. This can be estimated clinically by abdominal examination.
    B. Ultrasound measurement above 25 cm is considered abnormal.
    C. It tends to be excessive in twin-to-twin transfusion syndrome.
    D. It is reduced in renal agenesis.

Answer	

173. **Theme:** Investigation during pregnancy

Statements:

A. This is done under a direct ultrasound guide.
B. It is done between 16 and 20 weeks of gestation.
C. There is a 1.9% risk of pregnancy loss.
D. It is used to check for chromosomal abnormalities.

Answer	

174. **Theme:** Obstetrics assessment

Statements:

A. The diagonal conjugate measures the lower part of symphysis pubis to this area.
B. It is part of the posterior border of pelvic inlet.
C. It is prominent in the android type of pelvis.
D. It is easily palpable in a clinically inadequate pelvis.

Answer	

175. **Theme:** Obstetrics medical condition

Statements:

    A. It carries a risk of deteriorating retinopathy.
    B. The risk of pre-eclampsia increases three-fold.
    C. Poor control is associated with increased risk of congenital anomalies.
    D. Caudal regression syndrome has been attributed to this condition.

Answer	

176. **Theme:** Gynaecological malignancy

Statements:

    A. Histologically it demonstrates Psammoma calcification.
    B. Macroscopically it appears as a multiloculated cyst with papillary projections.
    C. Management includes debulking surgery followed by intravenous paclitaxel.
    D. This is the most common type of epithelial ovarian tumour.

Answer	

177. **Theme:** Obstetrics condition

Statements:

   A. This is caused by increased levels of melanocyte stimulating hormone and oestrogen during pregnancy.
   B. The incidence is 92 % in pregnant women.
   C. This is a dark line formed from the mid suprapubic area to the umbilicus.
   D. It usually disappears a few weeks after delivery.

Answer	

178. **Theme:** Abdominal incision

Statements:

   A. This is a transverse suprapubic incision.
   B. It has a low risk of herniation.
   C. It is less painful as few dermatomes are involved.
   D. It has limited accessibility.

Answer	

179. **Theme:** Congenital anomalies

Statements:

   A. This is complete gonadal dysgenesis.
   B. The streak gonad fails to produce hormones.
   C. The fetus is phenotypically female.
   D. The karyotype is XY.

Answer	

180. **Theme:** Abnormal vaginal bleeding

Statements:

   A. All patients with this condition should be investigated to rule out gynaecological cancer.
   B. It is commonly caused by atrophic vaginitis.
   C. It can be caused by unscheduled bleeding during hormone replacement therapy.
   D. Transvaginal ultrasound scan is done as an initial investigation for this condition.

Answer	

181. **Theme:** Drugs in Obstetrics and gynaecology

Statements:

A. This is used to induce abortion and medical management of miscarriage.
B. It is a prostaglandin analogue.
C. It can cause uterine tachysystole.
D. It can be inserted intravaginally or sublingually.

Answer	

182. **Theme:** Investigation in male subfertility

Statements:

A. A three-day sexual abstinence is advised before doing this test.
B. An abnormal test warrants a repeat three months later.
C. For a male with a very low count, hormonal profile (FSH, LH and testosterone should be performed.
D. Total count above 39 million per ejaculate is considered normal.

Answer	

183. **Theme:** Gynaecological procedure

Statements:

    A. This is recommended to be done three yearly.
    B. It is a screening test.
    C. Not routinely done above 65 years old.
    D. General advice is to avoid sex and douching for at least three days before the procedure.

Answer	

184. **Theme:** Antenatal monitoring

Statements:

    A. This is used to monitor patients with high risk of spontaneous preterm birth.
    B. It is best measured by transvaginal ultrasound.
    C. Progesterone (hydroxyprogesterone caproate) reduces the risk of preterm birth in women whose measurement is below normal.
    D. The combination of history and this examination can predict 80.6% of extremely early spontaneous preterm delivery.

Answer	

185. **Theme:** Risk factors for Obstetrics condition

Statements:

A. Multiple pregnancy.
B. Cervical weakness.
C. Infection.
D. Previous history of this condition.

Answer	

186. **Theme:** Drug in Obstetrics and gynaecology

Statements:

A. This is a progesterone antagonist.
B. It can be used together with misoprostol for termination of pregnancy.
C. It can reduce uterine fibroid size.
D. It can cause nausea, vomiting and diarrhoea.

Answer	

187. **Theme:** Management of endocrine gynaecological condition

Statements:

A. Eflornithine cream applied topically.
B. Cyproterone acetate alone or in combination with oestradiol.
C. Metformin.
D. Laser or electrolysis therapy.

Answer	

188. **Theme:** Management of early pregnancy complications

Statements:

A. Metoclopramide.
B. Fluid and electrolyte replacement.
C. Multivitamins.
D. Thromboprophylaxis

Answer	

189. **Theme:** Perianal area

Statements:

    A. It is supplied by branches from pudendal nerve.
    B. It is torn during third degree tear.
    C. Improperly repaired can result in fecal incontinence.
    D. Proper delivery technique can prevent its injury.

Answer	

190. **Theme:** Management of early pregnancy complications

Statements:

    A. Suction curettage.
    B. Serum Beta hCG follow up.
    C. Barrier method family planning.
    D. If hCG has reverted to normal within 56 days of pregnancy, follow up will be for 6 months from the date of evacuation.
    E. If hCG has not reverted within 56 days, then follow up will be 6 months after it normalizes.

Answer	

191. **Theme:** Risk factors for Obstetrics emergency

Statements: A. Prematurity. B. Breech presentation. C. Polyhydramnios. D. Oblique/transverse lie.	
Answer	

192. **Theme:** Risk factors for Obstetrics emergency

Statements: A. Positive previous history B. Gestational diabetic mellitus. C. Macrosomia. D. Instrumental delivery.	
Answer	

193. **Theme:** Congenital anomaly

Statements:

A. The ovary produces little or no sex hormone.
B. The problem may be with pituitary gland or hypothalamus.
C. There is a lack or delay of pubertal sexual maturation.
D. The treatment includes hormone replacement therapy.

Answer	

194. **Theme:** Management in Obstetrics emergencies

Statements:

A. Risk factors include retained placenta.
B. It can result in vasovagal shock.
C. Postnatally the uterus may not be palpable on abdominal examination.
D. The Hydrostatic (O'Sullivan) method can be used.

Answer	

195. **Theme:** Gynaecological procedure

Statements:

    A. It is indicated for Bartholin cyst or abscess.
    B. The less common alternative procedure is silver nitrate ablation.
    C. It is done under local, regional or general anaesthesia.
    D. The cyst is converted into a pouch.

Answer	

196. **Theme:** Female reproductive cycle

Statements:

    A. It can cause acute abdominal pain when ruptured.
    B. It is a temporary structure which appears monthly during reproductive cycle.
    C. On ultrasound the cyst appears thick walled with characteristics "ring of fire" peripheral vascularity.
    D. It produces progesterone.

Answer	

197. **Theme:** Perinatal event

Statements:

A. Abdominal ultrasound shows irregular overlapping of the cranial bones on one another (Spalding sign).
B. Ultrasound shows no fetal heart activity.
C. There are changes in the skin and tissues.
D. Wrinkled skin is the first and most obvious sign of this condition.

Answer	

198. **Theme:** Infection in Gynaecology

Statements:

A. It is easily treated with azithromycin or doxycycline.
B. There may be cervicitis with mucopurulent discharge.
C. Neonates born to an infected mother may develop conjunctivitis.
D. Nucleic acid amplification test is used for the diagnosis.

Answer	

199. **Theme:** Contraindication of hormonal therapy during menopause

Statements:	
A. Active liver disease. B. Known current venous thromboembolism. C. Breast cancer. D. Uncontrolled hypertension.	
Answer	

200. **Theme:** Side effects of hormonal treatment.

Statements:	
A. Fluid retention. B. Breast tenderness. C. Mood swing. D. Acne.	
Answer	

201. **Theme:** Benefit of hormonal treatment

Statements:

    A. Improvement of vasomotor symptoms.
    B. Increased bone mineral density.
    C. Low incidence and mortality of colon cancer.
    D. Improved sleep patterns.

Answer	

202. **Theme:** Management options in early pregnancy complication

Statements:

    A. Expectant management.
    B. Tablet methotrexate.
    C. Laparoscopic salpingectomy.
    D. Laparoscopic salpingostomy.

Answer	

ANSWERS

1	Primary dysfunctional labour
2	Yolk sac tumour
3	Dexamethasone / Betamethazone
4	Epidural / Spinal
5	Oxytocin
6	Paclitaxel
7	Testosterone
8	Serum ferritin
9	Cervical cancer stage 1b
10	Grand multipara
11	Hypothyroidism
12	Letrozole
13	Carboprost
14	Ovarian malignancy stage 1b
15	Placenta accreta spectrum (PAS)
16	Secondary arrest
17	Endometriosis
18	Artificial Rupture of Membranes
19	Neo adjuvant therapy
20	Monochorionic monoamniotic (MCMA)
21	Urinary Tract Infection
22	Oestrogen cream
23	Androgen insensitivity
24	Cervical ectropion
25	Congenital adrenal hyperplasia

26	Corpus luteum cyst (ruptured)
27	Colporrhaphy
28	Chancre
29	Mucinous cystadeno carcinoma
30	Germ cell tumour
31	IUGR
32	Amniotic fluid
33	Aneuploidy

34	Anhydramnios
35	Atociban
36	Gestational sac
37	Injectable progestogen
38	Neural tube defect
39	Secondary arrest of labour
40	Gastroschisis
41	Chicken pox
42	Patau syndrome
43	Endometrial hyperplasia
44	Fetal fibronectin
45	Rubella
46	Breech
47	Mullerian abnormalities
48	Macrosomia
49	Breech presentation
50	Parvovirus

51	Placenta
52	Propylthiouracil
53	Venous thromboembolism
54	Symphysis-fundal height
55	Toxoplasmosis
56	Duodenal atresia
57	Twin anaemia- polycythaemia sequence (TAPS)
58	Abdominal circumference
59	Yolk sac
60	Baseline variability
61	Laparoscopy
62	Clomiphene citrate
63	Baseline fetal heart rate
64	Mefenamic acid/ NSAIDS
65	5 alpha reductase deficiency
66	Tibolone
67	Functional ovarian cyst

68	Bimanual examination
69	LNG - IUS
70	Burch colposuspension
71	Imperforate hymen
72	Bacterial vaginosis
73	Dermoid cyst
74	Danazol
75	Endometrial ablation

76	Endometrial polyp
77	Endometriotic cyst
78	Cervical ectropion
79	Endometriosis
80	Levonogestrel intrauterine system
81	Caesarean hysterectomy
82	Carcinoma of cervix stage 1b
83	Fitz- Hugh-Curtis syndrome
84	Gardnerella vaginalis
85	Krukenberg tumours
86	Dyspareunia
87	Kallmann syndrome
88	Ovarian drilling
89	Lynch syndrome
90	Sertoli-Leydig cell tumours
91	Alpha methyl dopa
92	Primary peritoneal carcinoma
93	Endometrial cancer
94	Urodynamic testing
95	Tanner staging
96	Vulvodynia
97	Beta hCG
98	Vulva intraepithelial Neoplasia (VIN)

| 99 | Progesterone |
| 100 | HBA1C |

101	Oestriol
102	Cabergoline
103	Fortuitous
104	Sacral promontory
105	Ischial spine
106	Vasectomy
107	Breakthrough bleeding
108	Intermenstrual bleeding
109	Erythromycin
110	Folic acid
111	Cyproterone
112	Show
113	BRCA Gene
114	Nexplanon
115	Vaginal speculum
116	Precipitate labour
117	Chorioangioma
118	Calcium gluconate
119	Oestrone
120	Unstable lie
121	Postpartum blues
122	Choriocarcinoma
123	Uric acid
124	CEA
125	Indirect Coombs test
126	Acanthosis nigricans
127	Duodenal atresia
128	Kegel exercise
129	Liquor
130	Borderline ovarian tumour
131	Eisenmenger syndrome
132	Transverse lie
133	Conjoined twins
134	Retroverted uterus
135	Radiotherapy

136	Inguinal lymph nodes
137	Fresh frozen plasma
138	Internal iliac nodes
139	Proteinuria
140	Decidua
141	Low Grade Squamous Itraepithelial Lesion (LGSIL)
142	IVF
143	High Grade Squamous Intraepithelial Lesion (HGSIL)
144	Latent phase of labour
145	Leuprolide acetate
146	Mullerian agenesis
147	PCOS
148	Premature ovarian failure
149	SLE
150	Squamo-columnar junction
151	Hyperprolactinaemia
152	Endometrial cancer
153	Ovarian cancer
154	Fibronectin
155	Theca lutein cyst
156	Transformation zone
157	Anti-mullerian hormone
158	Insulin
159	Leuprolide acetate
160	Platelets concentrates.
161	Fetal growth chart
162	Metronidazole

163	Hyperemesis gravidarum
164	Cystocele
165	Fresh frozen plasma
166	Cryoprecipitate.
167	Exomphalos / Omphalocele
168	Chorioamnionitis
169	Human papilloma virus (HPV)

170	Omentum
171	Vasomotor symptoms
172	Liquor
173	Amniocentesis
174	Sacral promontory
175	Preexisting diabetes mellitus
176	Serous cystadenocarcinoma
177	Linear nigra
178	Pfannenstiel incision
179	Swyer syndrome
180	Postmenopausal bleeding
181	Misoprostol
182	Semen fluid analysis
183	Cervical smear
184	Cervical length
185	Preterm labour
186	Mifepristone
187	Hirsutism
188	Hyperemesis gravidarum
189	Anal sphincter
190	Gestational trophoblastic disease
191	Cord prolapses
192	Shoulder dystocia
193	Hypogonadotropic hypogonadism
194	Uterine inversion
195	Marsupialization
196	Corpus luteum
197	Macerated still birth.
198	Chlamydia trachomatis
199	Menopausal Hormone Therapy (MHT)
200	Progestogen
201	Menopausal Hormone Therapy (MHT)
202	Ectopic pregnancy

REFERENCES

1. Obstetrics by Ten Teachers / edited by Philip N. Baker 20th edition, London: Hodder Arnold, 2017

2. Gynaecology by Ten Teachers / edited by Ash Monga 20th edition, London: Hodder Arnold, 2016

3. Dewhurst's Textbook of Obstetrics & Gynaecology/ edited by D.Keith Edmonds 9th edition, Chichester,West Sussex: Wiley-Blackwell, 2018

3. Llewellyn-Jones Fundamentals of Obstetrics & Gynaecology edited by Jeremy Oats, Suzanne Abraham, 10th edition, Edinburgh/New York: Mosby/ Elsevier, 2015

www.ingramcontent.com/pod-product-compliance
Lightning Source LLC
Chambersburg PA
CBHW070121010626
45794CB00012B/709